APPLE CIDER
VINEGAR

TABLE OF CONTENT

1. INTRODUCTION

Apple cider vinegar also known as cider vinegar or ACV is a pale to amber color vinegar and is made from apple or cider. It is easy and quite in-expensive to make good quality organic, un-filtered and un-pasteurized apple cider vinegar at home level. Fermentation time will depend on the method chosen for making it. In one method the peels, cores and scraps are used. In the second method whole apples may be used.

Using the scraps peels and core method is beneficial in a way that allows you to enjoy your apple as well as utilize the waste to prepare high quality apple cider vinegar. It takes around two months for the apple cider vinegar to ferment from scraps and around six months from whole apples.

For centuries vinegars of many types have been used for many different purposes e. g. marinades, food preservatives, chutneys, salad dressings, meat tenderizer, cleaning, weed controlling, polishing, providing therapy for many ailments, as anti-septic, etc.

Recently apple cider vinegar has started regaining popularity as health supplement and health tonic. Few studies have suggested it to be beneficial in various conditions such as diabetes, obesity, hypertension, heart diseases, fighting infections, helping in digestion, increasing in food satiety value, relieving leg cramps, lowering serum cholesterol level, fighting bad breath, reducing chronic fatigue, reducing swelling, whitening teeth, killing foot fungus, fighting yeast infection, reducing heart burn, and so on.

Besides having many oral health benefits it has been well known to provide a wide variety of topical application functions and much beauty usage. It can be used as a facial toner, hair rinse, facial mask, bath soak, foot soak, sunburn treatment, age spot removal, deodorant, helps in getting rid of acne, relieves arthritis pain, use as a mouth wash, and so on.

The main contents of vinegar is acetic acid but it may contain other acids and vitamins, minerals, pectin (a soluble fiber), and amino acids, etc. All claims for its highly beneficial effects for all sorts of ailments are not proven through studies but many have ended in conclusion that it might have the potential for many unknown benefits. Besides acetic acid it also contains lactic acid, malic acid and citric acid.

Still few studies suggest that many claims made through experience of generations needed more in depth study to understand and fully utilize the unknown factual benefits hidden and the reasons behind its working. How it actually works inside a human body to benefit it needs better understanding through studies.

For commercial synthesis apples may be crushed to squeeze out the juice. Bacteria and yeast may be added to encourage alcoholic fermentation and its process. Sugar present in apples is turned into alcohol in this way. In the second half of the fermentation process, alcohol gets converted into vinegar by the action of bacteria called acetobacter which helps in the formation of acetic acid. Malic acid and acetic acid gives vinegar its sour taste. Conventional method of its production will need time and patience for the process of fermentation happening naturally. For large commercial production, quick processing methods may be applied to produce huge amounts of it in a short period of time.

There are also several other ways to produce apple cider vinegar on large scale for commercial purposes. Vinegar helps in adding the satiety of foods and a person who consumes it through meals experiences fullness for a longer period of time. It also reduces heart burn and regularizes bowel movement. It is also known to relieve chest congestion and boosts energy. It works as a blood thinner, provides relief from jelly fish sting pain, skin irritation, bug bite and aids in reducing blood pressure.

It provides more satiety of food and this may be a cause behind its association with weight loss besides other causes. According to the studies conducted in relation to vinegar with weight loss, it has been concluded that it might reduce body weight and obesity. More studies are needed to fully understand the working and relationship of it to weight reduction.

Very high intake for a long period of time may lead to hyper-reninemia, hyperkalemia and osteoporosis.

As apple cider vinegar is highly acidic its intake needed to be incorporated through dietary intake instead of isolated intake as direct intake causes skin burn due to it being highly acidic in nature. Even it can have burning effect on skin through outer application if applied in concentration.

More studies are needed in the area to fully understand the benefits of it and to segregate myths with facts in order to find the true value behind. It has been associated with providing natural remedies for many kinds of chronic diseases e. g. acid reflux, acne, constipation, weight loss, control of blood sugar, memory problems, reversing aging, etc.

ACV also acts like blood thinner and may also help in the prevention of high blood pressure. From during the time of Hippocrates it has been considered to be the father of all cures. During the wars it was being used as an antiseptic to treat the wounds. It is known to work as a natural detoxifying agent, providing relief from allergies, balancing the body pH, reducing inflammation and preventing flu.

How to incorporate it in our meals so that we can make the best use of it and ingest it in a way that gives us full potential of its benefits without overdosing it or taking it in isolation. Incorporating it in our meals to bring out the best possible results needs a real challenging situation. It is possible only by giving due consideration towards it and understanding the benefits attached to it by doing so.

Apples being highly nutritious fruit contain a wide variety of vitamins, minerals, amino acids, enzymes, pectin, etc. And in the making of apple cider vinegar apples are the main ingredients. All vinegars do not possess the same kind of natural remedial value as apple cider vinegar does. It also contains many enzymes, microbes and all the bye products produced during the processing.

It helps in purifying and detoxifying many body organs. It assists in oxidizing of blood, neutralizing toxic body substances and pathogenic bacteria, and promotes digestion and elimination process. There are also claims of it helping in the strengthening of the heart and anti-carcinogenic effects on certain types of cancers. Vinegar contains chromium which could have an altering effect on your insulin level.

Vinegar can be made from many fruits, vegetables and grains but apple cider vinegar as the name suggest is made from pulverized apples. No other vinegar possesses the same qualities as ACV. From being used as a folk remedy it has recently gained a more modern approach on its uses and benefits based on studies and researches.

ACV may also interact with medication for diabetes and heart diseases as well as with laxatives and diuretics. Food drug interaction needs to be understood fully by patients utilizing these medications for their treatment before starting on a new remedy.

You can make your own apple cider vinegar at home and can be sure of its quality and purity without having doubts that you might have about all the available commercial brands. Wash apples, dice them and put them in a glass jar. Do not remove peels and core. Fill water in the jar to cover the apples. Cover the jar with a piece of cloth or paper towel so that the oxygen can pass through it. Place the jar in a clean, dry, dark and warm place. Leave it to ferment for at least six months. Keep stirring it once a week for good results. After six months you will observe a layer of scum caused by bacteria on top of it. Filter the content with a cheese cloth. Let it stand for another 4-6 weeks for good results. Cover the jar and refrigerate it for longer storage.

2. PREVENTS STOMACH PROBLEMS

Apple cider vinegar has a natural bacteria fighting power and may contain magnesium, chlorine, phosphorus, potassium, sulfur, sodium, calcium, iron, copper and fluorine. It has been claimed to provide relief from indigestion problems, stomach churning, pain, acid reflux, constipation, heart burn, neutralizing toxic substances and bacteria, etc.

It can be added during food preparation for its consumption and can be used in moderate amounts on a daily basis to make full use of its therapeutic value and to improve the peristaltic movement of the gut. It is also known to flush out toxic waste from the body which helps in keeping the digestive system in peak condition.

One tea spoon full of it can be added in juices with honey to make a balanced drink. Besides it can also be added in soups, purees, gravies, sauces, salads, marinades and many more. Pickles, relishes and chutneys prepared from apple cider vinegar could be made a part of each meal to make a better use of it on a daily diet plan.

Use of ACV for health benefits helps in better making use of the natural remedies available which is being avoided and hindered by the pharmacological sector of any given society due to their vested interests strategic view.

For the relief of acid reflux, heart burn and nausea it has been recommended to add it to your drink with honey or in your soup 30 minutes or one hour before your meal. Within three days' time it has been claimed to relieve a person of all these symptoms.

3. CALMS DOWN DIGESTION

It helps in increased production of gastric juices and enzymes needed for proper digestion of each food eaten. These enzymes help in the breaking down of the food items into smaller and smaller pieces so that these valuable nutrients could be absorbed by the blood stream during digestion and benefits the body by providing nourishment whenever and where ever needed.

It also helps in increasing the acidity of food which is needed for digestion. Presence of pectin which is a soluble fiber must have a role to play in having a calming effect on digestion and intestinal spasm. Its antibiotic property can help in relieving diarrhea caused by bacteria.

The strong smell and typical strong taste of apple cider vinegar will be a little difficult to handle it in the beginning, but once you get used to it you can make it a regular part of your daily routine. To provide best natural remedies for your overall wellness and to make use of the great beneficial value provided by apple cider vinegar, it needs to be kept handy in your kitchen.

4. CLEARS NASAL CONGESTION

Apple cider vinegar helps in clearing the nasal congestion by steam inhalation. You may add it to your humidifier for the beneficial results and breathe it in. You may also add a little apple cider vinegar to a bowl and then pour boiling water in it. Start inhaling the steam till the water cools down. Repeating it twice or thrice daily can help you in getting relief from the symptoms in a natural way.

5. HELPS WITH HICCUPS

Hiccups usually lasts for a few minutes but at times may continue to last for a longer period of time which could be a cause of irritability and discomfort. Many natural remedies could be used to control it at home level before proceeding towards medical intervention or help. One such remedy is the use of apple cider vinegar in a drink to overcome it and to get relief from it. People have been trying it and have found it to be of substantially beneficial.

Take a cup of warm drinking water, add one tea spoon full of apple cider vinegar and two tea spoons full of honey in it, stir well and consume it sip by sip. If the problem persists for longer period of time than medical help may be advisable.

Hiccup is a repeated involuntary contraction of the diaphragm and in medical terminology is known as singultus or synchronous diaphragmatic flutter (SDF). Usually it is self-limiting and gets resolved without any intervention naturally. Apple cider vinegar can be tried initially as a natural home remedy. If the problem persists and gets chronic, medical attention may be considered.

6. SOOTHS YOUR SORE THROAT

Symptoms of sore throat can be treated successfully at home level through the use of apple cider vinegar appropriately. As apple cider vinegar has anti-bacterial properties it can help in fighting infections especially the one causing a sore throat. The pH of the tissues gets decreased by the acidity of the vinegar which helps in preventing bacterial growth on the surface. The presence of pre biotic inulin in raw ACV helps in increasing the number of white blood cells and T cells and boosts the immune system.

Consuming apple cider vinegar through a hot beverage and soups and sipping it twice or thrice daily can help in relieving sore throat. Adding a tea spoon full in your hot beverage or soup may help in soothing the symptoms. While resting after its consumption can bring out more beneficial results in shorter period of time.

Do not use apple cider vinegar more than one tea spoon at a time as it is acetic acid and could harm your tooth enamel if taken in excess or in high concentration. Taking one teaspoon full through a food medium is enough to bring out all the beneficial effects needed. Overdosing will not help in any way therefore patience is needed after you have used a natural remedy for your sore throat symptoms.

7. REDUCES SWELLING IN HANDS AND FEET

Natural home remedies are simple, tried and tested at home level, hassle free, in-expensive and easily approachable. Good use of common sense is needed when deciding upon when to use a simple natural home remedy and when to look for an expert's opinion. Serious medical condition need not be ignored.

In case of chronic medical condition do consult your medical practitioner before you use any kind of home remedy.

Swelling of hand and feet can be caused by fluid retention by the cells and tissues of the body and commonly referred to as edema. Edema can be a cause of pregnancy, PMS, high blood pressure, poor nutrition, menopause, cardiovascular diseases, cirrhosis of liver, kidney disease, swelling of the lymph nodes, etc.

Excessive intake of common salt in the diet may also help in retaining extra water in the body. It can also be caused by lack of potassium. The treatment needed to be based on resolving the underlying cause or causes of extra water inside the body leading to swelling. Apple cider vinegar is a natural home remedy that helps the body to remove extra fluids.

ACV can be consumed as mentioned earlier through a beverage or a soup. Only take a teaspoon full at a time once or twice daily. An apple cider vinegar soak can also benefit. Soak a piece of cloth in undiluted ACV and for at least fifteen minutes keep it wrapped around the swollen area. Another way to treat it is to immerse the affected area into one part ACV mixed with three parts of water. Besides possessing other active ingredients ACV also contain potassium which helps in relieving and treating symptoms of swelling naturally but not to the extent of relieving deficiencies. High potassium food sources needed to be added to avoid and to reverse the effects of deficiency if any.

8. REDUCES FATIGUE

Chronic fatigue can be a result of imbalanced dietary intake, stress, tension, lack of sleep and rest, dehydration and it can also be a cause of some underlying chronic condition or disease which needed to be investigated.

Release of lactic acid during exercising and prolong stress can cause fatigue. Apple cider vinegar helps in combating this with the help of its unique content of enzymes, potassium, amino acids and other substances. Drinking it through hot beverages and soups may help in relieving the symptoms gradually. Do not try to consume more than what has been recommended earlier. Also look towards the underlying causes of it and try to overcome these by properly eliminating the causes.

9. RELIEVES LEG CRAMPS

Leg cramps usually is not a serious problem but can be quite irritating and painful. There can be various underlying reasons behind this illness e. g. irregular muscle contraction, dehydration, electrolyte or mineral imbalance, etc. Low potassium level can also be a contributing factor leading towards these cramps especially the nocturnal type which you might be experiencing quite frequently.

Apple cider vinegar may help in overcoming the imbalances. One tea spoon full can be added to warm water with honey and can be taken twice or thrice daily to overcome this situation naturally. In addition to this eating foods that are high in potassium will help in overcoming the deficiency. Good food sources of potassium include banana, dried fruits, avocado, fresh mushrooms, milk and its products, tomatoes, potatoes, white beans, fish, squash, leafy green vegetables, etc.

Sodium in addition to potassium is responsible for maintaining the water balance in a human body. Consuming juices with a pinch of salt added can also help. Increasing your calcium and magnesium intake might also help. You may add a teaspoon full of apple cider vinegar with honey in your cocktail for effective results.

Drinking enough water and fluid is needed if the underlying cause is dehydration. You may also massage the affected area with undiluted ACV. Taking a hot bath and soaking the affected area may too benefit. Looking for the underlying cause and correcting the same will help in getting rid of the problem from its roots.

10. FIGHTS BAD BREATH

Halitosis or bad breath can be a sign of certain health problems. One of the common causes of it includes dental cavities, improper cleaning, cracked fillings, etc. Eating certain foods can also be a cause but which cannot and should not be avoided for its high nutritive value as these are essential for good health and wellbeing.

It can also be caused by bacteria feeding on food particles trapped in the mouth. Saliva production continuously provide natural cleansing ability and bad breath can also be a cause of xerostomia in which the mouth is dry due to lack of saliva production.

Many underlying diseases can also cause bad breath e. g. chronic bronchitis, constipation, diabetes, respiratory tract infection, liver disease, etc. Artificial and synthetic mouthwash can solve the problem temporarily and can contain substances that may be carcinogenic. Healthier, cheaper and natural substances can be used to overcome the problem without any side effects.

Adding one tea spoon full of each apple cider vinegar and honey to warm water, juice or cocktail and consuming it half an hour before meals can help in overcoming this problem naturally. Gargling after each meal with a diluted solution of ACV and water may also be effective.

It possesses a quality of being natural antibiotic and anti-septic which helps in fighting with these bad breath causing bacteria. It helps in increasing the secretion of saliva which will contribute as a natural cleanser. Good oral hygiene is a must in any case. Drinking too much coffee, sugary drink, alcohol and smoking can easily be avoided without affecting nutrition intake.

11. FIGHTS YEAST INFECTIONS

The natural acetic acid bacteria present in apple cider vinegar has the capability of fighting against yeast infection caused by Candida Albican. This yeast can cause infection in various parts of a human body e. g. gastric and esophageal lining, skin, mouth, etc. Through natural treatment of apple cider vinegar the growth of yeast is being restricted and hampered by good type bacteria.

The composition of ACV is such that it helps in boosting the body's immune system to fight against such infections. It could be consumed through a beverage, soup or through foods as well as could be applied on the affected areas with the help of a cotton wool or a piece of cloth. Rinsing your body with a diluted solution of vinegar and water for outer infection may also help.

You may need to consult a physician if you are unable to restrain the infection through natural therapy or if the infection seems to be spreading.

12. KILLS FOOT FUNGUS

A simple home remedy can help in getting relief from nail and toe fungus. ACV naturally possesses anti-fungal properties and it can provide a slow but definite cure for it. You will have to be patient for the result as fungal growth inside a nail is difficult to reach and cure. Other cure from medics may involve medication which every one might not be able to take. Surgical removal of the nail can be another option which many would like to avoid.

Apple cider vinegar could help in treating it naturally by oral intake as well as outer application to the affected area. Low sugar foods must follow this natural remedy. Without surgery or medication you will be able to get rid of it hopefully within a year's time naturally.

13. CONTROLS BLOOD SUGAR

According to the results of various studies conducted to understand the role of ACV in controlling blood sugar in diabetic patients is quite promising for its health benefits. Vinegar contains chromium which can alter the insulin level so medical advice is needed to be sought before starting to begin with this natural remedy.

If it is used in combination with diet and exercise it can help people with type 2 diabetes which is usually non-insulin dependent. It has been discovered that acetic acid the main constituent of apple cider vinegar inhibits the activity of many enzymes needed for carbohydrates digestion and absorption e. g. amylase, maltase, lactase and sucrase.

In the presence of ACV in the digestive tract a part of ingested sugars and starches will pass through without either getting digested or being absorbed by the blood.

14. INCREASES WEIGHT LOSS

Apple cider vinegar helps in losing weight by providing more satiety to foods as well as eliminating part of carbohydrates intake without being absorbed by the blood. More significant studies in the area are needed to fully understand the mechanism if any attached to the many claims being made.

15. LOWERS YOUR CHOLESTEROL

Apples are good source of soluble fiber like pectin. Apple cider vinegar primarily made from apples contains pectin which is a soluble fiber. Soluble fibers help in eliminating the dietary cholesterol instead of it being absorbed by the body by binding with it and getting excreted. It also helps in reducing the synthesis of cholesterol by the liver. Therefore it has been claimed to bring out the result of lowering serum cholesterol if taken in small amounts on daily basis especially through incorporation in meals.

16. USE AS A HAIR RINSE

Apple cider vinegar has several beauty benefits besides its many health benefits. It has great treatment effects if used as a hair rinse. It helps in the treatment of dandruff, hair loss, balancing scalp pH, removing various product buildup, etc. It also assists in improving the texture of hair and leaves them smooth, soft and shiny. It also aids in preventing split ends, dry scalp, frizz, tangles, etc.

It also assists in maintaining and replenishing the moisture of your hair. If used in combination with baking soda can work as a natural conditioner. The ideal pH for hair is slightly on the acidic side. Using the shampoos which are alkaline leaves the pH on the higher side. To bring it back to a lower side ACV rinse brings out the best results needed. It adds beauty, bounce and body to your hair naturally.

17. USE AS A FACIAL MASK

To give a finishing rinse to your face in order to cleanse it, treat it against microbes and to tighten the skin ACV facial mask can be used. It can also be used in combination with other beneficial ingredients e. g. honey. It should be applied over the face and left for treatment for at least 20 minutes. This mask could be used thrice weekly to bring out moisturizing and healing benefits as well as to maintain the pH of your skin. It can also be mixed with clay, or any of your favorite mask base to sooth and treat your skin once fortnightly or whenever needed especially in hot summer season.

18. TONE YOUR SKIN

Poor skin tone makes it appear uneven and older. Unbalanced dietary intake, over exposure to sunlight and aging can all contribute negatively to skin tone. To improve your skin tone you can utilize the beneficial effects of apple cider vinegar to control oil production, to give smooth texture and appearance to the skin and to clear blemishes.

It being a natural anti biotic also helps in reducing the breakouts caused by bacteria and yeast. Acids also help your skin to have more elasticity and keep it youthful for a longer period of time. As ACV is a natural product you do not have to worry about the chemical composition and harsh effects due to being synthetic.

It also improves blood circulation towards skin and gives it natural life and lift needed. To make a good toner, add equal amount of water and ACV in a bottle. Add few drops of your favorite oil and the toner is ready for application. Use it after washing your face by taking a little in your palm and applying it over your face. Repeat it 3 - 4 times weekly for good results.

19. USE AS A BATH SOAK

Apple cider vinegar bath soak can eliminate or reduce discomfort caused by sunburn. Add one cup of ACV to you bath and soak for at least 10 minutes to get relief from this discomfort. In order to recover from infection and inflammation this simple natural remedy will be beneficial. Also to detoxify your body you may avail the ACV bath soak. ACV can be used for detoxifying effects needed alone or in combination with other natural compounds.

It can be used for pain relief, to increase immunity, detoxification, sunburn, pain relief, athlete's foot, UTI, arthritis, etc. It also helps in maintaining the pH of the body and lowering stress related hormones. One cup of raw, unprocessed, organic apple cider vinegar can be added into warm bath. Half an hour of soaking the body in this solution will help in bringing out balancing changes needed.

20. WHITENS TEETH

Gargling with ACV in the morning may help in removing stains on teeth, whitens it and kills bacteria. Brush your teeth after gargling. For good result use it consistently for at least one whole month as nicotine and coffee stains are stubborn and difficult to remove.

Olive oil together with apple cider vinegar can be used as an alternative to a tooth paste for brushing your teeth for good results. ACV can also be used in isolation for the beneficial effects but do not use in excess or in saturation as it can damage the tooth enamel.

Besides using it as mouth wash or a tooth paste it needed to be taken orally through meals in a variety of ways to bring out best results. Many food items which are also helpful in whitening the teeth naturally include lemons, oranges, strawberries, carrots, broccoli, etc.

21. USE AS A FOOT SOAK

Apple cider vinegar can be used as a foot soak to get relief from foot odor, toe fungus, athletes foot, etc. It also helps in softening and soothing of dry skin and cracked heels. ACV foot soak can be used in many foot problems and conditions e. g. fatigued foot, warts, calluses, regular foot cure, etc.

Patients who are suffering from chronic diseases need to first consult their physician before starting on this home remedy especially people who have diabetes.

22. USE TO TREAT SUN BURN

Apple cider vinegar works well to treat and prevent sunburn by helping the skin to combat inflammation caused by it. To treat sunburn make use of diluted apple cider vinegar solution through a piece of cloth on the affected areas, let it dry and then spread a little amount of your favorite oil on it.

Follow this for a few days till it all heals up naturally. Sun burn can be quite discomforting caused due to excessive exposure to sunlight and may start showing signs within few hours which could range from mild to severe.

In severe condition medical intervention may be needed. It is better to avoid exposing skin to direct sunlight to prevent it to occur. Many synthetic sun blocks may contain chemical substances that can result in exposing your body to unnatural substances which may be a contributing factor in causing severe skin diseases and disorders.

23. GET RID OF AGE SPOTS

Application of apple cider vinegar on age spots with a piece of cloth or cotton helps in combating these naturally. Age spots are flat, brown or yellow discoloration of the skin and can occur on the hands, neck and face. These can be a cause of sun damage, improper liver function, nutrient deficiency, chronic constipation, lack of sleep, dehydration, lack of dietary intake of antioxidants, etc.

ACV can be applied in the diluted form as well as with many other combinations for better result. It can be used in combination with onion juice, sandal powder, rose water or olive oil.

24. NATURAL DEODORANT

After getting aware of all the harmful effects caused by much marketed and advertised varieties of deodorants and antiperspirant available in all the beautiful packaging, colors and shiny containers, one begins to start wondering about the alternatives and natural substitutes available.

Switching over to these natural remedies might need will power and tactics of simplifying through simple means instead of complicating it through synthetic means. Results of the uses of all sorts of synthetic living have started to show negative signs from all angles which could and should easily be avoided.

Many irreversible health damages could happen and therefore prevention is better than cure. Replacing all your artificial synthetic products with natural simple ones needs understanding of how each one works well. Apply diluted apple cider vinegar in place of synthetic deodorant for better overall results.

25. GET RID OF ACNE

The presence of acids in apple cider vinegar aids in ex foliating the dead cells, removing oil and fighting bacteria. Dab a piece of cloth in half strength solution of apple cider vinegar and water and apply it over your face giving special attention to the affected areas.

Green tea or your favorite oil can be added to get rid of the strong smell of apple cider vinegar. Having natural antibiotic properties it may help in killing bacteria causing this problem. It also helps in restoring the pH of our skin. How much time is needed for curing this will differ with each individual case.

Pure unfiltered apple cider vinegar can be used for this purpose. If you find the smell to be intolerable then apply only to the affected areas.

26. GET RID OF WARTS

Apple cider vinegar has been found to be successful in removing warts by people who have tried this home remedy. Warts are common dermatological problem which could be treated easily at home level with very low cost and without any side effects through AC V's proper application.

Warts are caused by viruses entering through cuts and breaks in the skin. Before going to bed soak a piece of cotton wool in ACV and keep over the wart and fasten it with Band-Aid. In the morning replace the old piece of cotton and Band-Aid with a fresh one. If it bothers you in the day time then only keep it at night time.

Keep repeating this for at least one week so that the chances of it re-appearing diminish and the problem gets solved from the roots.

27. RELIEVES ARTHRITIS PAIN

Topical application of apple cider vinegar mixed with olive oil and coconut oil can work wonders to relieve the pain of joints. Before going to sleep at night massage the effected painful areas of joint with this solution for at least ten to fifteen minutes. You can also apply heat after massage by resting the affected area on hot water bottle. Resting and sleeping is also very important.

Individual cases of arthritis may vary from each other. There are different forms of arthritis e. g.

juvenile arthritis, osteoarthritis, rheumatoid arthritis, septic arthritis, psoriatic arthritis, etc. Osteoarthritis is the most common form which is a degenerative disease of joints. Causes of osteoarthritis may involve age, infection of joints or it may be a result of trauma.

Major complaints may include persistent localized joint pain. It occurs due to inflammation around the joint and various other reasons. Apple cider vinegar benefits can also be availed to help reduce symptoms associated with joint pain by incorporating it through salads and dietary intake.

All varieties of fruits and vegetables are highly recommended for these patients to overcome the underlying causes. Best uses of fruits and vegetables which could be consumed in raw form needed to be made. Reducing weight by the intake of low calories and highly nutritious diet is needed. Increasing activity to tolerable degree is advisable to keep the joints in good working condition and to reduce weight if needed.

28. HELPS IN KILLING CANCER CELLS

Studies done to understand the role of apple cider vinegar to treat cancer patients have revealed certain facts that may be helpful in killing cancer cells or regressing their growth. But still no conclusive hypothesis is available currently to suggest any fact with guarantee.

ACV is acidic in nature but once inside the body it promotes the body towards increased alkalinity which is needed to treat cancer.

29. USE AS A MOUTH WASH

Apple cider vinegar in diluted form can be used as a mouthwash to combat bad breath as well as to provide anti septic properties once daily to help prevent cavities and infection and to cleanse your mouth.

Artificial and synthetic mouthwash contains many chemicals which have been found to be carcinogenic. In order to avoid these chemicals as they leave their residue in mouth, good use of better natural alternatives is needed.

30. CONCLUSION

After studying the benefits of apple cider vinegar at length we come to a solid conclusion that it needed to be made a part of dietary intake in whatever way it is feasible on a daily basis. It can be incorporated in a variety of ways while cooking and preparing meals for example, salads, soups, beverages, marinating of entree, casseroles, gravies, curries, breads, biscuits, etc.

Innovative ideas could be applied to create great recipes of interest and individual liking. People who like sour flavor would not find it hard to use it and apply it in their cookery methods and creations. Chinese cookery methods make high use of vinegar in their foods. Anyone who is fond of eating Chinese cuisine would also not find it difficult.

Vinegar also acts like a meat tenderizer. While cooking mutton, lamb or beef you may marinate the meat in apple cider vinegar for at least 3-4 hours before cooking to let the meat absorb its good sour flavor as well as tenderize it for easy cooking and also helping in lessening the time needed for meat to get tender. If you prepare it one day before and keep it refrigerated, it could bring out really good results.

Pickles, relishes and chutneys could easily be prepared at home level using apple cider vinegar and a variety of vegetables of individual likings and disliking. It need not be consumed in large amount as it is pure acid and needed to be used sparingly but regularly.

Besides meals it has many other beneficial uses from being as a house cleanser to a body cleanser. It has numerous other health and healing benefits. These simple home remedies helps in bringing simple ways and methods of doing things which helps in making living easier and worthy. In today's life of artificiality and modernization, people had been leaving behind the wisdom of the wise which need not be ignored or forgotten.

After we have become fully aware of the dangers of consuming synthetic chemicals in the form of medication even for simple health problems which could easily be resolved by good rest, sleep, eating pattern and living style. We have seen the results of the side effects these are causing not just to one person, or family, or community but in the global form.

People need to realize the importance of avoiding chemicals as much in their lives as possible not only in diet but all around their lives. Natural therapies and home remedies could wisely be applied as much as possible. Simple life makes it easier and even much cheaper with immeasurable benefits. The need only lies in realization of it and working towards it.

There are a wide variety of topical benefits attached with apple cider vinegar. These benefits may include soaking, massaging, gargling, brushing, toning, cleansing, disinfecting, treating, rinsing, etc. It can also be used with other natural substances to improve or increase its potency. Just be sure not to use any products for experimentation which might lead to many kinds of problematic situations.

Get well aware and use combinations that have been tried and tested. If you feel confident that you're created therapy works for you then do share it with others so that other people get well aware of it too. Responsible behavior towards this is needed as each ones wellbeing is others responsibility.

Do not use apple cider vinegar in concentration as it is quite potent, strong and harsh. Do use a base for some kind of dilution. Also do not be an extremist when it comes to dietary intake. Quick fixes by over dosing will only help in ruining your health and affecting it negatively. Patience is needed, and only think of it as a part of medication instead of part of a diet. As you are careful about not taking medications in excess so think the same way with ACV as it is no less than a medication when it comes to over dosing.

Think about it when in concentrated form it works like a meat tenderizer and when it goes inside your body in that saturated form what will happen inside. So never ever use it in saturation but use it as a salad dressing, flavor enhancer, meat tenderizer, and in many different ways in moderation that allows you to consume it as a part of meal and incorporated in your meal in small amounts. Concentrated forms of it might have a damaging effect on your tooth enamel, tissues and cells of your body and many unknown problems.

Use in concentrated form for outer application only as an anti-septic or to fight fungal growth and to treat warts. It can also be used as a treatment for insect bite, to reduce cellulite, fight infections, ease pain, and fade bruises, sooth bug bite and to relieve inflammation.

It is a very affordable and natural type of deodorant. Synthetic deodorants and antiperspirants act by blocking the sweating ability. Sweating is a natural body process to get rid of the toxins present inside. In this way it hinders the body's capability to detoxify. ACV gets absorbed and it helps in neutralizing the body perspiration odor.

ACV is acidic but once inside the body it promotes the body towards increased alkalinity which is a good sign for our health. It is also known to dissolve kidney stones. The best known fact about apple cider vinegar is its natural anti biotic properties and it is well known to possess anti-bacterial, anti-viral and anti-fungal properties.

ACV is also known to help relieve gout, gum infection, candida infection, sinus infection, ear infection, rheumatism, etc. It reacts positively with body toxins and helps in getting relief from them. But one thing is certain that no doubt it does possess numeral benefits to health and healing but cannot be a source of nourishment. People have been making it a part of food source which it cannot be. A very simple test at home level can prove it. Start boiling your ACV and evaporate all the water content of it. The total substance left in the end as residue is all the nourishment that it contains. Which you can see is negligible to the amount of nourishment that you need to take to stay healthy and well nourished. So please do not use it as a source of nourishment.

If you need potassium do look towards foods rich in potassium instead of believing ACV to overcome the deficiencies. It does contain a variety of nutrients but in insignificant quantity. Instead of calling it a tonic it needed to be called an antibiotic. Its antibiotic properties are much stronger and potent especially the outer application which cannot and should not be ignored.

Apple cider vinegar does not possess cure for all diseases. And the ones it has been promoted for do not possess solid scientific backing. Tried and tested by many as a successful home remedy for centuries it does not possess any obvious harmful effects known to us till now. Therefore trying it does not feature any side effects associated with it. Obviously over emphasizing its importance for all cures will lead to misguidance and various health risk factors.

It has been an ingredient of a part of cookery, medicine, beauty care, and many more. People have been mesmerized by much antibiotic potency it contains. Its true value need to be known and there is only one way of doing so is by finding facts about it through scientific research studies. Until this is done we know that it is only a natural substance and could be taken in moderation regularly without worrying about the side effects and negative cost to our health and wellbeing.